D0032539

*Quick*FACTS™

Advanced CANCER

What You Need to Know—NOW

QuickFACTS™

From the Experts at the American Cancer Society

Advanced
CANCER

What You Need to Know—NOW

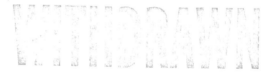

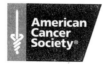

American
Cancer
Society®

Published by the American Cancer Society/Health Promotions
250 Williams Street NW, Atlanta, Georgia 30303 USA

Copyright ©2008 American Cancer Society

Printed in the United States of America
Cover designed by Jill Dible, Atlanta, GA

5 4 3 2 1   08 09 10 11 12

Library of Congress Cataloging-in-Publication Data

Quick facts advanced cancer: what you need to know now/
from the Experts at the American Cancer Society.
     p. cm.
  Includes bibliographical references and index.
  ISBN-13: 978-0-944235-68-3 (pbk.:alk. paper)
  ISBN-10: 0-944235-68-9 (pbk.:alk. paper)
  1. Cancer—Popular works. I. American Cancer Society.
RC263.Q53 2008
616.99'4—dc22

                           2006016979

A Note to the Reader

This information represents the views of the doctors and nurses
serving on the American Cancer Society's Cancer Information
Database Editorial Board. These views are based on their
interpretation of studies published in medical journals, as well
as their own professional experience.

The treatment information in this book is not official policy of
the Society and is not intended as medical advice to replace the
expertise and judgment of your cancer care team. It is intended
to help you and your family make informed decisions, together
with your doctor.

Your doctor may have reasons for suggesting a treatment plan
different from these general treatment options. Don't hesitate to
ask him or her questions about your treatment options.

For more information, contact your American Cancer Society
at **800-ACS-2345** or **http://www.cancer.org.**

Bulk purchases of this book are available at a discount.
For information, contact the American Cancer Society at
trade.sales@cancer.org.

Table of Contents

Treatment

Your Advanced Cancer

Introduction

Advanced cancer* is not well defined. Doctors diagnose advanced cancer based on several factors:

- how much cancer is present
- how far the cancer has spread
- how much the cancer has affected your physical condition
- whether there is any effective treatment for your cancer

Some people believe that if **cancer** has spread to other parts of the body (called **metastatic cancer**), it is the same as advanced cancer. This is not necessarily true. You can have widespread cancer, but it can still be treatable and sometimes curable. Examples of this are testicular cancer and certain types of **leukemia** and **lymphoma.** On the other hand, your cancer may not have spread to distant sites and still be considered advanced because there is too much cancer to be removed

*Terms in **bold type** are further explained in the Glossary, beginning on page 83.

or because it has caused major health problems for you. An example of this is pancreatic cancer. You may not be sure if you have advanced cancer. Even if you do have advanced cancer, some parts of this book may not apply to you.

This book addresses some of the problems and solutions associated with advanced cancer. It is intended to help you better understand what advanced cancer is, what can be expected if it happens, and what you can do about it. Discuss any questions or concerns you may have with your **cancer care team.** They are best able to help you understand your specific situation, as well as your cancer type, stage, treatment, and outcomes.

What Is Advanced Cancer?

Advanced cancer, generally, is cancer that has spread beyond the organ where it first started. Often it has spread widely throughout the body (called metastatic cancer). Advanced cancer is not always metastatic cancer (see the section "How Is Metastatic Cancer Different from Advanced Cancer?" page 5). But metastatic cancer may be considered advanced if it is affecting a vital organ and cannot be removed.

The term advanced cancer usually means that the cancer cannot be cured. Even if there is no cure, however, treatment may help shrink the cancer, relieve symptoms, and extend your life. Some people can live for many years with advanced cancer.

Every person's cancer is unique. Your cancer may respond differently to treatments and grow at a different rate than the same cancer in someone else. For some people, the cancer may already be advanced when they first learn they have the disease. In other people, advanced cancer develops after years of treatment. In general, advanced cancer usually occurs after you have had cancer for some time and treatment is no longer effective in stopping its growth. The symptoms often related to advanced cancer, like pain and depression, almost always continue to respond to treatment.

What Is Metastatic Cancer?

Metastatic cancer is cancer that has spread from the part of the body where it started (its **primary site**) to other parts of the body. When cells break away from a cancerous **tumor,** they can travel to other areas of the body through either the bloodstream or lymphatic channels.

If the **cancer cells** travel through lymphatic channels they can become trapped in **lymph nodes,** often those closest to the cancer's primary site. If the cells travel through the bloodstream, they can go to any part of the body. Most often, the cancer cells break off and travel in the bloodstream. Most of these cells die, but occasionally they don't. They can settle in a new location, begin to grow, and form new tumors. The spread of a cancer to a new part of the body is called **metastasis**.

Even when cancer has spread to a new location, it is still named for the part of the body where it started. For example, if prostate cancer spreads to the bones, it is still called prostate cancer, and if breast cancer spreads to the lungs it is still called breast cancer. When cancer comes back in a patient who appeared to be free of cancer (in **remission**) after treatment, it is called a **recurrence.** Cancer may recur in several ways:

- **local recurrence,** in or near the same organ in which it developed;
- **regional recurrence,** in nearby lymph nodes or in the area from which lymph nodes had been removed; or
- **distant recurrence,** involving any other part of the body not included in local or regional recurrence. Distant recurrence is also called **metastatic recurrence.** For example, the cancer might recur in parts of the body away from the primary site, such as in bones, the liver, or the lungs. This happens because some cancer cells have broken off from the original tumor, traveled elsewhere, and begun growing in these new places.

Sometimes metastatic tumors have already developed when the cancer is first diagnosed. In some cases, metastasis may be discovered before the primary (original) tumor is found. If a cancer has spread widely throughout the body before it is discovered, it may be impossible to determine exactly where it started. This condition is called

cancer of unknown primary. To learn more about this condition, contact the American Cancer Society at **800-ACS-2345.**

What Is Recurrent Cancer?

Recurrence is a medical word that means the cancer has come back in a patient who appeared to be free of cancer (in remission) after treatment. Cancer can come back

- in the same organ or **tissues** where it started or in nearby tissues;
- in lymph nodes near the original cancer; or
- in distant organs.

How Is Metastatic Cancer Different from Advanced Cancer?

Metastatic cancer is not necessarily the same as advanced cancer. Cancer is called metastatic even if only a small amount of the cancer has spread. In many cases, metastatic cancer can be treated successfully if it has not already done a lot of damage. Sometimes if only a small number of tumors are present, they can be surgically removed and the patient cured. Metastatic cancer may be advanced if it has spread to many places in the body or has greatly harmed tissues and important organs.

Most people who die of cancer have metastatic tumors. Many of the problems caused by cancer occur because the cancer has spread to an area of the body that is very important to survival or because the cancer has spread to many areas.

Risk Factors and Causes

Do We Know What Causes Metastatic Cancer?

How Cancer Cells Spread

Metastasis is the end result of a multistep process. Cancer cells travel from the organ in which they develop through the blood and/or lymphatic vessels to other parts in the body.

Step 1 is the development of some cancer cells that are faster growing and more likely to spread. The cancer cells in a tumor are not all the same. As the cancer grows, some of the cells that develop are more "**malignant**" than others. These are cells that grow faster and also tend to spread.

Step 2 is **angiogenesis.** This is when the tumor promotes the development of its own blood vessels and blood supply so that it can grow faster.

Step 3 is the growth of the more malignant cells that tend to spread. Normal cells that make up organs such as the lungs and liver are held in place by a substance called **extracellular matrix** or **ECM.** This is like the mortar holding bricks together to form the walls of buildings. For cancer to spread, its cells must break loose from the ECM. Cancer cells may do this by producing enzymes that break down the ECM. Breaking loose from a tumor is only the first of many steps a cancer cell must take before it can spread. Cancer cells also undergo changes that enable them to break through the walls of blood vessels or lymphatic vessels and get into other tissues.

Step 4 is survival in the bloodstream. Most of the tumor cells entering the blood or lymph circulation are destroyed by natural immune system responses. Only the most malignant cells will survive.

Step 5 is the ability of the cells, once they have survived, to attach to distant organs or lymph nodes.

Step 6 is a key part of growth in a new environment—the ability of the new tumors to form new blood vessels (a process called angiogenesis) that carry nutrients and oxygen to the growing tumor.

Step 7 is the ability of these cancer cells to grow in their new environment and avoid the body's attempts to reject or destroy them.

Why Cancer Cells Tend to Spread to Certain Parts of the Body

The type of cancer and where it starts often determines where it will spread. Most tumor cells that have been dislodged from the original tumor are carried in the blood or lymphatic circulation until they get trapped in the next "downstream"

capillary bed or lymph node(s). This explains why breast cancer often spreads to axillary (underarm) lymph nodes but rarely to lymph nodes in the groin. Likewise, the lung is a common site of metastasis for many cancers. This is because the heart pumps blood from the rest of the body through the lung's blood vessels before sending it elsewhere. The liver is a common site of metastasis for cancer cells arising in the stomach and intestines because blood from the intestines flows into the liver.

Doctors have learned that cancer cells often break away from the main (primary) tumor and circulate in the blood. Usually they don't settle in any particular organ, and they eventually die. When the cancer does spread to other organs, it is because of certain genetic changes in the cells. Scientists are beginning to recognize these changes, and someday they may be able to look for them to determine whether a person's cancer is the type that will spread to other organs. Research is also being done that focuses treatment on blocking or targeting the genetic changes so the cells cannot spread and grow.

Sometimes the patterns of metastasis (or spread) cannot be explained by anatomy. Some cancer cells are able to find and invade specific sites. This "homing" pattern may be caused by specific substances on the surfaces of cancer cells that stick to the cells in certain organs. In other cases, cells of some organs release hormone-like factors that actually cause cancer cells to grow faster.

Which Cancers Spread Where?

Following is a brief description of where specific cancers are likely to spread. For more information on these cancers, refer to the American Cancer Society documents for these cancer sites.

Bladder

Bladder cancer tends to grow locally and invade local tissues such as the pelvic wall. It also spreads to the lungs, liver, and bone.

Brain

Brain cancer rarely spreads outside the brain. It mainly grows throughout the brain.

Breast

Breast cancer most commonly spreads to the bone but also can spread to the liver, lung, and brain. As the cancer progresses, it may affect any organ, even the eye. It can also spread to the skin near where the cancer started.

Colorectal

The most common site for colon cancer to spread to is the liver. The next sites are bone and lung. Spread to the brain is uncommon.

Rectal cancer commonly spreads to the lung, brain, and bone. Its major site of spread is in the pelvis, where the rectal cancer started. This can be painful because it can grow into nerves and bones in this area.

Esophageal

Esophageal cancer mostly grows locally. As it progresses, swallowing may become difficult. This can occur suddenly or gradually over several months.

Kidney

Kidney or renal cancer can grow locally and invade surrounding tissues. When it spreads, the lungs and bones are the most common sites.

Leukemia

Leukemias advance by filling the **bone marrow** with leukemia cells. The normal bone marrow is replaced and cannot produce normal cells, such as oxygen-carrying red cells, infection-fighting white cells, or platelets that stop bleeding.

Liver

Liver cancer doesn't often spread outside the liver; rather, it grows in the liver as it becomes advanced.

Lung

Lung cancer can spread to any organ of the body, but most often it will spread to the liver, bones, and brain. It will grow in the lung and spread to other parts of the lung. It can also grow into the sac around the heart (**pericardium**).

Lymphoma

Lymphomas tend to stay in the lymph nodes and bone marrow. They will spread to other organs when they are very far advanced. The involvement of lymph nodes can be very troublesome because this can cause fluid to accumulate in the abdomen and lungs, as well as in the arms and legs.

Melanoma

Melanoma can spread anywhere in the body. It first tends to go to local lymph nodes but then can spread through the blood to the brain, lungs, liver, and bone.

Mouth and throat

Cancers of the mouth, throat, or nasal passages tend to grow locally. When they spread, it is usually to the lungs.

Multiple myeloma

Multiple myeloma mainly stays in the bone where it started and rarely spreads elsewhere. But myeloma cells produce substances that cause the bones to weaken and fracture. Because it dissolves bones, the release of so much calcium causes hypercalcemia. Myeloma protein produced in large amounts can damage the kidneys. This reduces a person's ability to dispose of excess salt, fluid, and body waste products. Myeloma patients are about 15 times more likely to develop infections than are healthy people. The most common and serious of these is pneumonia.

Ovarian

Ovarian cancer, in the advanced stage, most often spreads to the lining and organs of the abdomen and can cause a buildup of fluid and swelling in the abdomen. It can also spread to the outer lining of the lung and cause fluid to accumulate there. It much less often spreads outside the abdomen and pelvis.

Pancreatic

Pancreatic cancer mainly stays in the abdomen and grows locally, as well as spreading to the liver. It can also spread to the lungs, bones, and brain.

Prostate

Prostate cancer, when it spreads, usually goes to the bones. Much less often, it will spread to other organs, including the brain.

Stomach

Gastric or stomach cancer tends to spread locally and within the abdomen. The next areas it goes to are the liver and lungs. Spread to the bone and brain is less common.

How Many People Get Advanced Cancer?

More than half a million people will develop and die of advanced cancer each year in the United States. Over 70% of these people will be older than age 65. Although more than 60% of all people who get cancer will live 5 years or longer, people with advanced cancer usually live less than 1 year.

Prevention

Can Advanced or Metastatic Cancer Be Prevented?

The only sure way to prevent the spread or growth of a cancer is to find the cancer early enough and remove it or destroy it. The American Cancer Society recommends early detection tests for cancers of the breast, cervix, prostate, and colon and rectum. But many people either do not know about or do not follow these recommendations and are more likely to have cancer discovered after it has already spread. Early detection tests are not perfect. Some cancers may spread before they can be found. Many cancers cannot be found early by any of the tests now available.

Researchers are looking for ways to keep cancer from spreading. For example, drugs are being studied that might block the **enzymes** that help cancer cells break through the walls of blood vessels. Other drugs block the formation of new blood vessels. Some patients, such as those with breast or colorectal cancer, are given drugs after surgery to kill cancer cells that might have broken away from the primary tumor.

Diagnosis

How Is Advanced Cancer Found?

It is hard to know who will develop metastatic or advanced cancer. Some cancers are more likely to spread than others. One way to predict this is to compare how closely the cancer cells resemble normal cells (called **grade**). The more normal the cells look, the less likely the cancer will spread. Another way of determining whether the cancer will spread is related to the size of the tumor. Also, if the cancer is found to have spread to nearby lymph nodes, it is much more likely to spread to distant sites. This is sometimes discovered after surgery if lymph nodes are removed and examined under the microscope.

Even when these things are known, doctors aren't always sure if a person's cancer will spread or whether he or she already has advanced cancer. Most of the time, the doctor will look at the patient's history and perform a physical examination. The patient will also have some blood tests and **imaging tests.** Taken together, this information helps the doctor determine whether the cancer is advanced.

Signs and Symptoms

Below are some **signs** and **symptoms** of advanced cancer and ways it is diagnosed.

The most telling symptom is loss of energy and **fatigue** (feeling tired). Most people with advanced cancer have a hard time doing everyday tasks. They often need help. At some point, it gets so bad that they spend much of their time in bed. Weight loss is another sign.

Pain may go along with advanced cancer, but this is not always the case. **Dyspnea,** or shortness of breath, may also occur.

For more about symptoms, please see the section "Managing Physical Problems of Advanced Cancer," pages 38–51.

Physical Examination

Along with asking about your symptoms, your doctor can learn much from examining you. These are some of the signs of advanced cancer:

- fluid in the lungs or in the abdominal cavity
- tumor lumps on or within the body
- an enlarged liver

Blood Tests

Certain blood tests can point to advanced cancer. Test results of liver function are often abnormal if the cancer has invaded the liver. Your cancer might produce a substance called a **tumor marker.** Examples of tumor markers are **prostate-specific antigen (PSA)** for prostate cancer or **carcinoembryonic antigen (CEA)** for colon cancer. The level of these substances in the blood may be very high. There are many other tumor markers for other cancers. For more information, see the American Cancer Society document *Tumor Markers,* available at **www.cancer.org** or by calling **800-ACS-2345.**

Imaging Tests

Chest x-ray

A chest **x-ray** can help detect tumors in your lungs or fluid in your chest.

Computed tomography

Computed tomography, commonly known as a **CT scan,** is an x-ray procedure that produces detailed cross-sectional images of your body. Instead of taking one picture, like a conventional x-ray, a CT scanner takes many pictures as it rotates around you. A computer then combines these pictures into an image of a slice of your body. The machine will take pictures and form multiple images of the part of your body that is being studied. Often, after the first set of pictures is taken, you will receive an **intravenous** (IV) injection of a "dye" or contrast agent that helps better outline structures in your body. A second set of pictures is then taken.

CT scans can also be used to guide a biopsy needle precisely into a suspected metastasis. For this procedure, called a **CT–guided needle biopsy,** the patient remains on the CT scanning table while a **radiologist** advances a biopsy needle toward the location of the mass. CT scans are repeated until the doctor is confident that the needle is within the mass. A **fine needle biopsy** sample (tiny fragment of tissue) or a **core needle biopsy** sample (a thin cylinder of tissue about 1/2 inch long and less than 1/8 inch in diameter) is removed and examined under a microscope.

CT scans are more tedious than regular x-rays. They take longer and you usually need to lie still on a table for 15 to 30 minutes while they are being done. But just like other computerized devices, CT scanning is getting faster. Also, you might feel a bit confined by the equipment in which you have to lie while the pictures are being taken.

You will need an IV line through which the **contrast dye** is injected. The injection can also cause some flushing. Some people are allergic to the contrast dye and get hives or, rarely, people have more serious reactions like trouble breathing and low blood pressure. Be sure to tell the doctor if you have ever had a reaction to any contrast material used for x-rays. You may also be asked to drink 1 to 2 pints of a contrast solution. The contrast solution helps outline the intestine so that it is not mistaken for a tumor.

Magnetic resonance imaging

Magnetic resonance imaging (MRI) scans use radio waves and strong magnets instead of x-rays. The energy from the radio waves is absorbed and then released in a pattern formed by the type of tissue and by certain diseases. A computer translates the pattern of radio waves given off by the tissues into a very detailed image of parts of the body. Not only does this produce cross-sectional slices of the body like a CT scanner, it can also produce slices that are parallel with the length of your body. A contrast material might be injected just as with CT scans, but this is done less often.

MRI scans are also very helpful in looking at the brain and spinal cord. MRI scans are a little more uncomfortable for the patient than are CT scans. First, they take longer—often up to an hour. Also, the patient has to be placed inside tube-like equipment, which is confining and can create anxiety for those who have a fear of enclosed spaces. When undergoing this procedure, try keeping your eyes closed to stay calm. Think of pleasant, relaxing images to make the time pass quickly. Feel free to ask for anti-anxiety medicines if you think they will help you. Finally, if you have a strong fear of enclosed areas, you can look for a facility that has an open MRI (one without an enclosed tube). Many cities have at least one MRI center that has an open MRI.

The MRI machine makes a thumping noise like a washing machine that you may find annoying. Some places provide headphones with music to block this out. Most people have little trouble managing the MRI experience. However, you should feel free to discuss any concerns you may have with your doctor or nurse. While you are undergoing the MRI, you will be able to talk to the technician throughout the procedure.

Positron emission tomography

Positron emission tomography (PET) uses a form of sugar (glucose) that contains a radioactive atom. A special camera can detect the radioactivity. Cancer cells absorb high amounts of the radioactive sugar because of their high rate of metabolism. PET is useful when your doctor thinks your cancer has spread but doesn't know where. A PET scan can be used instead of several different x-rays because it scans your whole body.

Ultrasound

Ultrasound is the use of sound waves to make images of internal organs. The computer displays the image on a computer screen. Ultrasound is useful for finding out whether some tumors are cancerous. This is a very easy test to take, and it uses no x-rays. You just lie on a table while someone moves a flat wand over your skin.

Radionuclide bone scan

A **radionuclide bone scan** helps show whether a cancer has metastasized to bones. You will be given an intravenous injection of radioactive material called **technetium diphosphonate.** The injection itself is the only uncomfortable part of the scanning procedure. The amount of radioactivity used is low compared with the much higher doses used in **radiation therapy,** and this low level of radiation does not cause any **side effects.**

The radioactive substance is attracted to diseased bone cells throughout the entire skeleton. Areas of diseased bone are seen on the **bone scan** image as dense gray to black areas called **hot spots.** These areas may suggest that metastatic cancer is present, but arthritis, infection, or other bone diseases can also cause hot spots. The pattern of these other diseases is usually different from the pattern caused by cancer. To distinguish among these conditions, the cancer care team may use other imaging tests or take bone biopsies. Bone scans can help detect metastases much earlier than regular x-rays. Not only are they useful in spotting bone metastases, they can also track how they respond to treatments.

Sometimes bone scans do not reveal areas of spread to the bones. This happens most often with **osteolytic metastases,** which destroy or dissolve bone. In some patients, the scan may show no radioactivity in certain areas of bone that have been totally destroyed by the cancer.

Biopsy

When an imaging test reveals something that is not normal, the doctor will want to be certain about whether it is cancer. This is usually determined by taking a small piece of tissue and looking at it under the microscope. This procedure is called a **biopsy.** Usually, a biopsy is performed by inserting a needle into the spot and extracting fluid, fragments of tissue, or a core of tissue. These samples are then examined under the microscope. It is important that your doctor is certain whether the cancer has spread, and often a biopsy is the only way to know for sure.

Treatment

How Is Advanced Cancer Treated?

Goals of Treatment

Advanced cancer is not likely to be cured, but it can often be controlled. The physical symptoms can almost always be well managed. At any stage of cancer, the goal of treatment should be clear to both you and your family. You should know whether the goal is to cure your cancer, extend your life, or relieve symptoms. This can sometimes be confusing because some treatments used to cure cancer may also be used to relieve symptoms.

Some people believe that nothing more can be done if the cancer cannot be cured. And so they stop all treatment. There are even doctors who think this way. Radiation, chemotherapy, surgery, and other treatments can often control symptoms. Relieving symptoms like pain, blocked bowels, upset stomach, and vomiting can help keep you more comfortable. Something can always be done to help maintain or improve your **quality of life.**

You have the right to be the decision maker in planning your treatment. The goal of any cancer care is to give you the best possible quality of life. This is a very personal issue. You should tell the cancer care team what is important to you. Tell them what you want to be able to continue to do.

Some people decide that burdens placed on them by aggressive cancer treatments are not worth the small chance of benefits. They may decide that they no longer want aggressive treatment. Others want to continue cancer treatments. Some patients want to stay at home. Others choose to go to an assisted living center, a nursing home, or an inpatient **hospice** program. Again, you should make the choices that you feel are best and most realistic for you and your situation.

You may decide that you don't want any more treatment for your cancer. This may be hard for some of your loved ones to accept, but you have the right to make this decision. Still, it is always best to include your family in difficult decisions.

Treatment choices for advanced cancer depend on where the cancer started and if and how much it has spread. As a general rule for cancer that has spread, **systemic therapy** such as **chemotherapy** or **hormone therapy** is required. Systemic therapy is treatment that is taken by mouth or injected into the blood to reach cancer cells throughout the entire body.

Surgery

In cancer treatment, surgery is generally used for cancer that is localized. Most of the time, the intent of surgery is to cure. Sometimes, for a localized cancer, surgery may be used to remove only the major part of the tumor, leaving other treatments such as radiation and chemotherapy to get rid of the rest. If the cancer has spread to only one area and is not large, then it may be possible to remove it completely. For example, if cancer has spread to the liver and there are only 3 or 4 tumors, then it may be possible for the tumors to be removed surgically.

Surgery is not often used in treating advanced cancer. But sometimes surgery can be helpful, as in the examples given below.

Surgery to relieve symptoms and improve your quality of life

Surgery can improve your quality of life and may even help you live longer, even when cancer has spread too far to be cured with surgery. For example, cancer can sometimes block the bowel (intestine). A surgeon may be able to bypass the blockage so the bowel can work normally again. In other cases, it may be necessary to let the bowel drain outside the abdomen into a bag (**colostomy**). Sometimes, simple surgery is used to put feeding tubes in place or to place smaller tubes into blood vessels for giving medicines to relieve pain.

Surgery to stop bleeding

Surgery may be done if there is a lot of bleeding from the stomach or bowel. To find the site of bleeding, doctors will usually look inside the intestinal tract, either from the mouth or rectum, with a flexible fiberoptic tube. This is done while the patient is sedated. The doctor may be able to stop bleeding by electrical **cauterization** of the bleeding vessel. If this cannot be done and if the patient is agreeable, surgery to close the blood vessel or remove the part of bowel that is bleeding may be the next step.

Surgery to stop pain

Sometimes a tumor may be pressing on a nerve or be too close to the spinal cord. Either cutting the nerve or removing the tumor may relieve the pain or prevent paralysis. When doctors operate on pancreatic cancer, they will often cut the nerves that cause pain in the pancreas.

Surgery to prevent broken bones

Cancer may weaken bones, causing fractures (breaks) that tend to heal very poorly. An operation to insert a metal rod can prevent some fractures if the bone looks weak. This usually occurs in the thigh bone. If the bone is already broken, surgery can rapidly relieve pain and help you be more active.

Whether surgery will help depends on your physical condition. Major surgery is hardly ever successful if you are bedridden. The stress of the surgery can set you back even further. On the other hand, surgery may be a good idea if you are feeling fairly well and are active.

Radiation Therapy

Radiation therapy uses high-energy x-rays to kill cancer cells. Radiation therapy can sometimes cure cancer that has not spread too far or too much. In advanced cancer, radiation therapy is often used to shrink tumors to reduce pain or other symptoms (called **palliative radiation**).

External beam radiation therapy is like a regular x-ray procedure except it lasts a little longer. Patients usually have treatments 5 days a week for up to 3 weeks. Sometimes, the number of trips for treatment can be reduced to just 1 or 2 days a week by giving more radiation during each session.

The main side effects of radiation therapy are fatigue (tiredness) and skin that may feel slightly sunburned. Radiation to the head and neck area can damage the glands that make saliva and cause a sore throat or mouth sores. Some people have trouble swallowing or lose their ability to taste food. Radiation to the stomach area can cause nausea, vomiting, diarrhea, and possible damage to the intestines. Radiation to the chest area may result in scars in the lungs that may cause shortness of breath in some people. Brain radiation can sometimes cause problems with thinking or memory that start several months to years after treatment.

Internal radiation therapy, or **brachytherapy,** uses small seeds of radioactive material placed directly into the cancer. The seeds can deliver a lot of radiation to a small area and spare the normal tissue around it.

Some radioactive materials such as strontium-89 (Metastron) can be given into a vein. They are drawn to areas of bone that contain cancer. The radiation given off by the drug kills cancer cells and relieves bone pain, but it will not cure cancer.

If there has been metastasis to many bones, this may work better than only using external beam radiation that only treats a small area. Sometimes different types of radiation are used together.

Chemotherapy

Chemotherapy uses anticancer drugs that are usually injected into a vein or taken by mouth. These drugs enter the bloodstream and go throughout the body, making this treatment useful for cancer that is widespread. In many cancers, chemotherapy can shrink tumors. This generally makes you feel better and can reduce any pain you might have. Chemotherapy can even prolong life in some patients with advanced cancer.

Drugs used in chemotherapy kill cancer cells, but they can also harm some of the normal, healthy cells in your body. This can cause various side effects:

- nausea and vomiting
- loss of appetite
- hair loss (hair grows back after treatment ends)
- mouth sores
- increased chance of infection
- bleeding or bruising after small cuts or injuries
- fatigue (tiredness)

Your cancer care team can suggest many steps to ease side effects. For example, there are drugs to help reduce nausea and vomiting. Sometimes it will help for the doctor to change the dose or the time of day you take your medicines. It is important to balance these side effects against the symptoms you are trying to relieve.

Hormone Therapy

Estrogen, a hormone made by women's ovaries, promotes growth of many breast cancers. Likewise, **androgens** (male sex hormones) such as testosterone, which is made by the testicles, promote growth of most prostate cancers. Drugs can be given that will block the action of these hormones or reduce the amount that is made. Side effects depend on the type of hormone treatments used. These side effects may include hot flashes, blood clots, and loss of sex drive.

Bisphosphonates

Bisphosphonates are a group of drugs used to strengthen bones that have been weakened by osteoporosis. Some of these drugs, such as pamidronate disodium (Aredia) and zoledronic acid (Zometa), are used to treat patients with cancer that has spread to and weakened their bones. Bisphosphonates are also used to treat cancers that start in the bones, for example, multiple myeloma. They help reduce bone pain and slow down bone damage caused by the cancer. These drugs are most effective when x-rays show the metastatic cancer appears to be causing the bone to become thinner and weaker. They are less effective when the cancer causes the bone to become denser.

Bisphosphonates can cause problems, however. Some patients develop damage to their jawbone, which can be quite painful. This seems to happen most often in patients who have had dental work while taking the drugs. More information on this topic can be found in the American Cancer Society book *QuickFACTS™ Bone Metastasis.* You can obtain this book through the Web site: **www.cancer.org/bookstore**.

Clinical Trials

The purpose of clinical trials

Studies of promising new or experimental treatments in patients are known as **clinical trials.** A clinical trial is only done when there is some reason to believe that the treatment being studied may be valuable to the patient. Treatments used in clinical trials are often found to have real benefits. Researchers conduct studies of new treatments to answer the following questions:

- Is the treatment helpful?
- How does this new type of treatment work?
- Does it work better than other treatments already available?
- What side effects does the treatment cause?
- Are the side effects greater or less than the standard treatment?
- Do the benefits outweigh the side effects?
- In which patients is the treatment most likely to be helpful?

Types of clinical trials

There are 3 phases of clinical trials in which a treatment is studied before it is eligible for approval by the **U.S. Food and Drug Administration (FDA).**

Phase I clinical trials

The purpose of a phase I study is to find the best way to give a new treatment and to determine how much of it can be given safely. Doctors watch patients carefully for any harmful side effects. The treatment has been well tested in laboratory and animal studies, but the side effects in patients are not completely known. Doctors conducting the clinical trial start by giving very low doses of the drug to the first patients and increasing the dose for later groups of patients until side effects appear. Although doctors are hoping to help patients, the main purpose of a phase I study is to test the safety of the drug.

Phase II clinical trials

These studies are designed to see if the drug works. Patients are given the highest dose that doesn't cause severe side effects (determined from the phase I study) and closely observed for an effect on the cancer. The doctors also look for side effects.

Phase III clinical trials

In phase III studies, promising new agents are scientifically compared with standard treatments. Phase III studies involve large numbers of patients. Some clinical trials enroll thousands of patients. One group, the **control group,** receives the standard (most accepted) treatment. The other groups receive the new treatment. Usually doctors study only 1 new treatment to see if it works better than the standard treatment. Sometimes they will test 2 or 3 at the same time. All patients in phase III studies are closely watched. The study will be stopped if the side effects of the new treatment are too severe or if one group has had much better results than the others.

If you are in a clinical trial, you will have a team of experts taking care of you and monitoring your progress very carefully. The study is especially designed to pay close attention to you.

There are some risks. No one involved in the study knows in advance whether the treatment will work or exactly what side effects will occur. That is what the study is designed to discover. Most side effects disappear in time, but some can be permanent or even life threatening. Keep in mind that even standard treatments have side effects. Depending on many factors, you may decide to enroll in a clinical trial.

Deciding to enter a clinical trial

Enrollment in any clinical trial is completely up to you. Your doctors and nurses will explain the study to you in detail and will give you a form to read and sign indicating your desire to take part. This process is known as giving your **informed consent.** Even after signing the form and after the clinical trial begins, you are free to leave the study at any time, for any reason. Taking part in the study will not prevent you from getting other medical care you may need.

To find out more about clinical trials, talk to your cancer care team. These are some of the questions you should ask:

- Is there a clinical trial for which I would be eligible?
- What is the purpose of the study?
- What kinds of tests and treatments does the study involve?
- What does this treatment do?
- Will I know which treatment I receive?
- What is likely to happen in my case with, or without, this new research treatment?
- What are my other choices and their advantages and disadvantages?
- How could the study affect my daily life?
- What side effects can I expect from the study? Can the side effects be controlled?
- Will I have to be hospitalized? If so, how often and for how long?
- Will the study cost me anything? Will any of the treatment be free?
- If I am harmed as a result of the research, to what treatment would I be entitled?
- What type of long-term follow-up care is part of the study?
- Has the treatment been used to treat other types of cancers?

The American Cancer Society offers a clinical trials matching service for patients, their family, and friends. You can gain access to this service through the National Cancer Information Center (**800-ACS-2345**) or by visiting this Web site:

http://clinicaltrials.cancer.org. Based on the information you provide about your cancer type, stage, and previous treatments, this service can compile a list of clinical trials that match your medical needs. In finding a center most convenient for you, the service can also take into account where you live and whether you are willing to travel.

You can also get a list of current clinical trials by calling the National Cancer Institute's (NCI) Cancer Information Service toll free at **800-4-CANCER** or by visiting the NCI clinical trials Web site: **www.cancer.gov/clinical_trials/**.

Complementary and Alternative Methods

Complementary and alternative therapies are diverse health care practices, systems, and products that are not part of usual medical treatment. They may include products such as vitamins, herbs, or dietary supplements, or procedures such as acupuncture and massage. There is a great deal of interest today in complementary and alternative treatments for cancer. Many are now being studied to find out if they are truly helpful to people with cancer.

You may hear about different treatments from family, friends, and others, which may be offered as a way to treat your cancer or to help you feel better. Some of these treatments are harmless in certain situations, whereas others have been shown to cause harm. Most of them are of unproven benefit.

The American Cancer Society defines **complementary medicine** or methods as those that are used along with your regular medical care. If these treatments are carefully managed, they may add to your comfort and well-being.

Alternative medicine is defined as methods or treatments that are used instead of your regular medical care. Some of them have been proven not to be useful or even to be harmful, but are still promoted as "cures." If you choose to use these alternatives, they may reduce your chance of fighting your cancer by delaying, replacing, or interfering with regular cancer treatment.

Before changing your treatment or adding any of these methods, discuss this openly with your doctor or nurse. Some methods can be safely used along with standard medical treatment. Others can interfere with standard treatment or cause serious side effects. That is why it's important to talk with your doctor. More information about specific complementary and alternative therapies used for cancer is available through our toll-free number or on our Web site.

More Treatment Information

For more details on treatment options—including some that may not be addressed in this document—the National Comprehensive Cancer Network (NCCN) and the National Cancer Institute (NCI) are good sources of information.

The NCCN comprises experts from 21 of the nation's leading cancer centers and develops cancer treatment guidelines for doctors to use when treating patients. Those are available on the NCCN Web site (**www.nccn.org**).

The American Cancer Society collaborates with the NCCN to produce a version of some of these treatment guidelines, written specifically for patients and their families. These less technical versions are available on both the ACS Web site (**www.cancer.org**) and the NCCN Web site (**www.nccn.org**). To receive a print version of these guidelines, call **800-ACS-2345.**

The NCI provides treatment guidelines via its telephone information center (**800-4-CANCER**) and its Web site (**www.cancer.gov**). Detailed guidelines intended for use by cancer care professionals are also available on **www.cancer.gov.**

Managing Physical Problems of Advanced Cancer

This section describes the major problems that can arise from advanced cancer. You may have some of these problems and symptoms or none of them. The following section, "Problems According to Cancer Site," describes problems related to specific types of cancer.

Broken Bones (Fractures)

When cancer invades bones, it can weaken them and sometimes lead to fractures, particularly in the leg bones near the hip. That is because these bones support most of your weight. You may have very bad pain for a while before the fracture occurs. An x-ray may show that the bone is likely to break before a fracture happens.

Treatment

The best treatment is to prevent the fracture. This is done through surgery. Surgeons place a metal rod through the weakened part of the bone. They do this while you are asleep under general **anesthesia.**

If the bone has already broken, then something else will be done to support the bone. Usually surgeons place an external steel support over the fracture.

External beam radiation may also be given to prevent any further damage by the cancer. Usually about 10 to 15 treatments are needed, although some doctors give the total dose of radiation in only 1 or 2 treatments. The radiation therapy will not strengthen the bone, but it may stop further damage. Surgery will still be needed to prevent a fracture.

Medicines or the cancer itself may cause confusion, dizziness, or weakness, which can lead to falls and accidents. Falls can cause fractures, especially to bones weakened by the cancer. Talk with your cancer care team about safety equipment you can use at home. Some things that you might find helpful are shower chairs, walkers, and handrails.

Blocked Bowel (Bowel Obstruction)

When cancer blocks either the small intestine or large intestine (colon), digested food cannot move through. This is called bowel obstruction. The symptoms include severe cramping, pain in the abdomen, and vomiting. The vomit may contain digested food and bile. Bowel obstruction occurs most often with abdominal or pelvic cancers.

Treatment

It is very hard to solve obstruction with surgery, and many patients are too sick to handle surgery. Others have such a poor outlook that surgery may not help much. Most studies have shown that patients with advanced cancer who develop this problem live only a short time. The decision to have surgery should be weighed against the chances of returning to a comfortable life.

An operation called a colostomy may help if only the colon is blocked. In this operation, the surgeon cuts the colon above the blockage. The cut end is then brought to the outside of the abdomen. Your stool can empty into a bag that is put around the opening.

Treating only the symptoms is often the best choice for many patients. This is called supportive care. For example, doctors may remove the stomach's contents through a tube placed through your nose and attached to a suction device. This often relieves nausea and vomiting. The next step would be for you to stop eating and to drink only small amounts to relieve thirst. You can take medicines for pain and nausea as a shot (injection) or as a patch.

Fatigue (Tiredness)

Fatigue is one of the most common symptoms reported by cancer patients. It is a physical, mental, and emotional tiredness that is not relieved with rest. It can make it hard for you to find the energy to do the things you normally do. Fatigue can be caused by these factors:

- the cancer itself
- the cancer treatment
- not eating well
- pain
- feeling depressed
- not enough **red blood cells** (anemia)

Treatment

There is no one cure for fatigue. In each case, treatment is aimed at the cause of the fatigue.

Blood transfusions can help some patients who have **anemia** (low red blood cell counts). Other patients can take medicines that help the body make more red blood cells. Talk with your doctor about treatments for severe anemia.

Light or medium exercise with a lot of rest breaks in between can often help with fatigue. You can also save energy by doing what needs to be done first and letting other things wait. Try to think of energy as gold. You want to invest only in what's most important to you. Spread your activities all through the day rather than trying to get things done all at once.

Sometimes stimulant drugs can help to overcome the feelings of fatigue. This is a possibility you may want to discuss with your cancer care team.

Unfortunately, doctors haven't yet explained why the cancer itself causes fatigue. It may be caused by natural substances called **cytokines.** The body produces these substances in response to the cancer, much as they are produced in the course of an infection such as influenza.

For more information, please see the booklet *Cancer-Related Fatigue: Treatment Guidelines for Patients.* To make sure you have the most recent guidelines, go to the American Cancer Society Web site (**www.cancer.org**) or call **800-ACS-2345.**

Hypercalcemia (Too Much Calcium in the Blood)

Cancer patients may have **hypercalcemia** (too much calcium in their blood) for many reasons. Most often, it is related to cancer that has spread to the bones. This causes calcium to be released from the bones into the bloodstream. Other times the cancer cells make a substance that causes high calcium levels. Blood levels of calcium can get so high that it is dangerous.

Early symptoms of too much calcium include the following:

- constipation
- passing urine very often
- feeling sluggish
- feeling thirsty all the time and drinking large amounts of fluid

Late signs and symptoms are coma and kidney failure.

Treatment

Giving fluids and certain drugs (pamidronate disodium and zoledronic acid) can quickly bring blood calcium down. These are usually given into the veins by intravenous (IV) infusion.

If the cancer can't be treated, the problem will come back and you will have to treat the blood calcium problem again. Sometimes a high blood calcium level can be the first sign of cancer, and treatment of the cancer will also treat the calcium problem.

Nausea and Vomiting

Advanced cancer can cause nausea and vomiting, either from radiation or chemotherapy treatments or from the cancer itself. Nausea and vomiting are most commonly caused by the treatments, and they generally get better over time after treatment is finished.

Nausea and vomiting are problems for many cancer patients, especially with treatment. In a small number of cancer patients, just thinking about getting their cancer treatments can make them feel nauseated. There is effective treatment for this problem.

Too much vomiting can be dangerous. It can cause **dehydration** (losing too much water) or **aspiration** (breathing food or liquids into the lungs).

Treatment for nausea

- Try bland foods, such as dry toast, crackers, Popsicles, gelatin, or cold clear liquids.
- Eat several small meals and snacks at bedtime if you get sick only between meals.
- Eat things that smell pleasant, such as lemon drops or mints.
- Eat food cold or at room temperature to make the smell and taste weaker.

- Ask the doctor about medicines to help with nausea.
- Try to rest quietly with your head elevated for at least an hour after each meal.
- Learn meditation and relaxation techniques.
- Distract yourself with soft music, a favorite TV program, or company.

Treatment for vomiting

- If you are in bed, lie on your side so that you won't breathe in or swallow your vomit.
- Sometimes taking a medicine by mouth (orally) can bring on nausea or vomiting. Ask the doctor to prescribe your medicines as suppositories. (Suppositories are drugs that can be administered through the rectum. The medicine in the suppository is absorbed into the bloodstream and then travels to the brain to stop the nausea.)
- Learn meditation, self-hypnosis, and relaxation techniques.
- Eat ice chips or frozen juice chips that you can munch on slowly.

Things to avoid

- Don't force yourself to eat or drink when you have an upset stomach.
- Don't lie flat on your back.
- Stay away from foods that have strong smells.
- Don't eat foods that are sweet, fatty, salty, or spicy.
- Stop eating for 4 to 8 hours if you are vomiting a lot. After that time, try clear liquids.

Call the doctor if you experience any of the following:

- breathe in or swallow vomit
- throw up more than 3 times an hour for 3 hours or longer
- see blood or something that looks like coffee grounds in your vomit
- can't keep down more than 4 cups of liquid or ice chips in a day
- can't eat for more than 2 days
- can't take your medicines
- feel weak or dizzy

The American Cancer Society has more information on how to manage nausea and vomiting. Call **800-ACS-2345** and ask for *Nutrition for the Person with Cancer: A Guide for Patients and Families* and *Nausea and Vomiting Treatment Guidelines for Patients with Cancer.*

Pain

There are many ways to ease pain caused by cancer. Sometimes pain is relieved by treatments that kill cancer cells (such as chemotherapy or radiation therapy) or slow their growth (such as hormone therapy or bisphosphonates). Don't be afraid to use medicines or other treatments, including complementary therapies, to help with your pain. Getting effective pain relief will help you feel better. It will make it easier for you to focus on the things that are important in your life. Some studies show that cancer patients who get effective pain treatment may live longer than those who do not. The first and most important step is letting your cancer care team know about your pain.

Treatment

Medicine taken by mouth is the most common way to treat pain. Often 2 or more drugs are used together. Other ways to help with pain include massage, heat and cold, and changing your body position.

Usually your doctor will start with drugs such as acetaminophen (Tylenol) or nonsteroidal anti-inflammatory drugs such as ibuprofen (Motrin). If these aren't helping, you will likely be given an opioid such as codeine, hydrocodone, morphine, or oxycodone. Codeine and hydrocodone are considered "mild" opioids, while morphine and oxycodone are stronger. Opioids are considered the best drugs for helping cancer patients control their pain. Unless you have a history of drug or alcohol abuse, you can take these drugs without worrying about getting addicted. Discuss any of your concerns with your doctor or nurse. It is rare for cancer patients to develop an addiction to opioids.

With all pain medicines, it is very important that you take the medicine regularly for these reasons:

- to maintain enough of the medicine in your bloodstream to keep your pain controlled
- to prevent the pain from becoming so bad that you will have to take more pain medicine than you normally do to get the pain controlled

Opioids can make you drowsy. They can also cause nausea and constipation. Most of the drowsiness usually goes away after a few days. It may not go away if you are taking high doses. You may have to choose between having less pain and being drowsy or having more pain and being more alert. The constipation can be helped by regular use of stool softeners, fiber, laxatives, drinking plenty of liquids, and being active.

The best treatment for you depends on the type of pain you are having and how bad it is. Tell your cancer care team if the methods you are using are not working.

Doctors have learned that not all patients respond to pain medicines the same way. Some medicines work better for some patients while others are less effective. Research has shown that this may be related to small genetic differences among people. This means that if one pain medicine, particularly an opioid, isn't helping you, it may be worthwhile to try a different opioid.

Also, some people require much higher doses of opioids than others. Do not be concerned about needing to take large amounts of drugs. It has nothing to do with your being intolerant of pain or a "complainer." It just means that your body needs more medicine than average.

The American Cancer Society has more detailed information on how to manage pain. Call **800-ACS-2345** and ask for *Pain Control: A Guide for People with Cancer and Their Families* and *Cancer Pain Treatment Guidelines for Patients.*

Paralysis Due to Pressure on the Spinal Cord

Cancer sometimes spreads to the bones in the spine. As the tumor grows, it can put pressure on the nerves in the spinal cord. Symptoms can range from pain to weakness and paralysis (not being able to move). This also can affect the nerves to your bladder so you will have trouble urinating. Early treatment can help reduce permanent nerve damage.

Symptoms to watch for
- trouble passing urine
- numbness or weakness of the legs
- very bad pain in the middle of your lower back

Tell your doctor right away if you have these symptoms. An MRI can usually reveal whether the cancer is pressing on your spinal cord. This is considered a medical emergency, and treatment should begin promptly.

Treatment
- steroids (prednisone or dexamethasone) to reduce swelling and treat pain
- radiation therapy to shrink the tumor that is causing the problem
- surgery to remove all or part of the tumor

Skin Problems

People with long-term illnesses often get skin problems from sitting or lying too long in one position. Cancer patients may also get skin problems from not eating well, not being able to move around, swelling, and some cancer treatments.

Treatment

Talk with your cancer care team. They can recommend a skin care program for your special needs. The most important things you can do are to change positions often when you are sitting or lying down and to keep your skin clean and dry.

Superior Vena Cava Obstruction (Blocked Blood Flow to the Heart)

The superior vena cava is the main vein that returns blood to the heart from the upper body. This vein runs through the upper middle chest. Pressure from tumors in the chest or lung can block the blood flow in this vein, causing blood to back up in the lungs, face, and arms.

Symptoms include the following:

- shortness of breath
- a feeling of fullness in the head
- swelling in the face and arms
- coughing
- chest pain

Treatment

Radiation therapy and/or chemotherapy can help shrink the tumor. If this is not possible, you may have a metal tube (stent) placed in the vein. This tube is inserted through a large vein in your arm or neck and then threaded through the obstruction.

Dyspnea (Trouble Breathing)

Dyspnea (trouble breathing) can be caused by a tumor blocking the airway or by a buildup of fluid around the lungs. Some patients with a very low red blood cell count (severe anemia) may also feel short of breath. A tumor blocking blood flow to the heart is another possible cause (see "Superior Vena Cava Obstruction" on page 49).

Treatment

When it is possible, treating the cause will help relieve shortness of breath. Sometimes external beam radiation or laser treatment (given through a bronchoscope) can shrink a tumor in the lung.

Patients with fluid around the lungs may feel better after having this fluid removed. After numbing the skin, the doctor places a needle into the chest and drains the fluid.

Oxygen is very helpful. It is given through a little tube that goes under the nose.

Opioids like morphine are the most helpful drugs to relieve the feeling of shortness of breath. Anti-anxiety medicines, like diazepam (Valium) can also help.

Having trouble breathing can make you feel anxious, worried, and even like you are going to panic. Some patients find these complementary methods helpful to relieve anxiety related to breathing difficulties:

- relaxation methods
- biofeedback
- guided imagery
- therapeutic touch
- aromatherapy
- music and art therapy
- distraction (watching movies, television, reading)
- a fan blowing air on you

Weight Loss and Not Eating Well (Poor Nutrition)

As cancer gets worse, many people feel weak, lose their appetite, and lose a lot of weight. The reason for these effects is not known, but here are some possible causes:

- substances released by the cancer into the blood
- inability to absorb nutrients from food

Treatment

It is very hard to treat these problems. Feeding through an intravenous (IV) tube rarely helps. It can burden patients with needles, tubes, and other supplies. Feeding through a stomach tube is also uncomfortable and rarely helpful.

Sometimes, the best thing you can do is to eat smaller amounts more often. Avoid low-calorie or low-fat foods. This is the time for high-calorie foods and liquids.

Two drugs are helpful in improving appetite. One is megestrol acetate (Megace). The other is dronabinol (Marinol). Drugs that help the stomach empty, such as metoclopramide (Reglan), can also help improve your ability to eat.

Problems According to Cancer Site

This section talks about the symptoms you might have when cancer spreads to different places in your body. Not everyone will get all the symptoms. Some of the information may not apply to you. Your doctor can tell you the most about your condition. Be sure to have regular checkups to find and treat the spread of cancer.

Treatment is covered briefly in this section. For more about treatment for a given symptom, see the section, "Managing Physical Problems of Advanced Cancer," pages 38–51.

Cancer Spread to the Abdomen

When fluid has collected and built up in the abdomen, it is called **ascites.** This extra fluid can make your belly expand and cause discomfort. It can also make it hard to breathe.

Treatment

The doctor removes the fluid through a needle. This relieves the problem for a while, but it will likely come back.

Cancer can spread to the bowels and cause blockage (obstruction). This causes very bad cramping and vomiting. If the cancer has only spread to the colon (large intestine), surgery may help.

Treatment

Colostomy or bypassing the blockage with surgery can help, if you are strong enough to have surgery. This is explained on pages 39–40 under "Blocked Bowel."

Cancer can also spread to or block the thin tubes (ureters) that carry urine from the kidneys to the bladder. If this happens, you may stop passing urine. Also, you will feel very tired and sick to your stomach.

Treatment

A tube can be threaded through the ureters to allow urine to flow again.

Cancer Spread to Bones

Your main symptom will be pain where the cancer is. Even though the cancer may have spread to many places in the bone, it usually hurts in only a few. Sometimes a bone will weaken and break. This happens with bones that support your weight, like the leg bones. But it can also happen to the bones of the back. The first symptom may be a sudden very bad pain in the middle of your back. See "Broken Bones" on pages 38–39.

Treatment

- drugs that strengthen bones (bisphosphonates)
- radioactive compounds, such as strontium-89, that are given into a vein
- radiation therapy to an especially painful bone

Preventing broken bones

- Stay away from activity that is hard on your bones (examples: heavy lifting, jogging).
- Any very weak bone may need a protective rod put in by a bone surgeon.

Cancer Spread to the Brain

The most common symptom is a headache or losing movement in part of your body, like an arm or leg. The other common symptom is sleepiness. You may have problems with other things, too. These can include hearing, eyesight, confusion, and even passing urine.

Treatment

Radiation treatment is best for these symptoms. Cortisone-like drugs, such as dexamethasone, can often help with symptoms.

Seizures are another symptom of cancer in the brain. They aren't common. But they can be very upsetting and scary both to you and to those around you.

Treatment

Medicines called anticonvulsants can prevent seizures.

Cancer Spread to the Liver

You may lose your appetite and feel tired. Some patients feel pain in the upper right part of the abdomen, where the liver is located. Usually the pain is not bad and is less of a problem than the tiredness and appetite loss. If there is a lot of cancer in the liver, your skin may turn yellow. This is called **jaundice.**

Treatment

- If there are fewer than 4 to 5 tumors, they can sometimes be treated by cryotherapy (freezing), surgery, or radio waves.
- For more tumors, chemotherapy may help. This may be given into a vein or directly into a blood vessel leading to the liver.
- **Embolization** (plugging up the blood supply) to the cancer with Gelfoam may help.

See also treatment information for your specific symptoms in "Managing Physical Problems of Advanced Cancer," pages 38–51.

Cancer Spread to the Chest or Lungs

The cancer may cause fluid to build up around the lungs. This can make you short of breath. (Also see "Dyspnea" in the section, "Managing Physical Problems of Advanced Cancer," pages 49–50.)

Treatment
- removal of fluid that has built up around the lungs through a needle
- chemotherapy and hormone therapy
- external radiation therapy
- surgery
- placement of a chemical or talc in the space to prevent further fluid buildup

The cancer itself can cause shortness of breath and chest pain as it spreads to more and more lung tissue.

Treatment
- oxygen
- opioids, such as morphine, for pain

The cancer can also spread to one of the large tubes that air passes through as it goes into your lung. This will make you short of breath. The lung may even collapse because it isn't being filled up as you breathe.

Treatment
- Laser treatment may partially remove the tumor.
- Radiation therapy may shrink the tumor.

The cancer can also grow into the pericardium, the sac surrounding the heart. This is not common, but it can cause fluid to build up around the heart. Symptoms include shortness of breath, low blood pressure, swelling of your body, and feeling tired.

Treatment

Removing the fluid with a needle can provide relief. This usually is done in a hospital setting because the heartbeat needs to be monitored. Often this procedure is followed with radiation and/or putting a chemical into the pericardium that prevents further fluid buildup.

Cancer Spread to the Skin

You will have lumps on the skin. Usually this does not cause symptoms. Sometimes breast cancer can come back in the skin over the chest and get infected. The open sores that result can smell bad.

Treatment

- Radiation treatment to the sores can shrink them and dry them out. This can only be done if you haven't had any radiation treatment before.
- Certain chemotherapy drugs can be put directly on the tumors and help dry up the sores.
- **Antibiotics** can help take away the smell. The antibiotics may either be pills or an ointment put directly on the sores.

Questions to Ask

What Should You Ask Your Doctor About Your Cancer?

It is important to have open and honest communications with your doctor about your condition. Your doctor and the rest of the cancer care team want to answer all of your questions. Have a family member or a friend with you during discussions. Take notes or ask if you can record the conversation.

Consider these questions:

- What treatment choices do I have?
- Which treatment do you recommend, and why?
- Is this treatment intended to cure the cancer, to help me live longer, or to relieve or prevent symptoms of the cancer?
- What side effects are likely to result from the treatment(s) that you recommend, and what can I do to help reduce these side effects?
- Where can I get a second opinion before I start treatment, and would a second opinion be helpful to me?

Coping

Coping With Advanced Cancer

Advanced cancer can be very scary and may be the hardest problem you and your family have ever faced. If you and your family have ongoing concerns that interfere with your lives, or if you simply want to maximize your communication and coping, you should talk with a licensed mental health professional. Being able to talk with an expert about your unique situation may bring you a great deal of comfort. **Social workers, psychologists,** and **psychiatrists** are all licensed mental health professionals who can be located through your **oncologist** or through the nearest large hospital in your area. Even one session with a licensed mental health professional can help you and your family focus on what matters most in your lives at this time. Your oncologist will be happy to work with you to find the right professional for you.

Dealing with Worry and the Unknown

Learning that you have advanced cancer may make you feel lost and afraid. This is natural. You may have questions such as these:

- What is going to happen to me?
- Have I done everything I should have done?
- What are my other options?

- Am I going to die?
- How much control will I have over my own life?
- Will my wishes be followed?
- How much pain and suffering will I have?
- What if I feel that I can't take much more treatment?
- How can I burden my family in this way?
- Will this be too much for my family to bear?
- What am I going to do about money?
- How long am I going to have to go through this?
- What happens when I die?

The list of fears may be overwhelming even to think about, much less experience. Worrying may make it hard for you to focus. You may even have tight muscles, trembling, and shakiness. Restlessness, shortness of breath, heart racing, sweating, dry mouth, and grouchiness are other signs of worry. Few people have all of these symptoms. Fortunately, there are professionals who can help you manage these concerns. In addition to your doctor and nurse, there are social workers, psychologists, psychiatrists, and pastoral counselors who are specially trained to help you talk about your concerns, control your fears, and make meaning of the experience. They are also available to support your family. Your doctor will know the local mental health experts in your community.

Likewise, a loved one may have similar feelings in his or her role as caregiver, money manager, spouse, child, or breadwinner. They may benefit from seeing a mental health professional as well.

Managing worry
- Talking about feelings may help relieve worry. Choosing the right person to talk with can be important. For some, that person will be a minister or a best friend. For others, it will be a family member.
- Trying to relax with deep breathing and relaxing body postures can be helpful. It works best if you practice and do it regularly.
- Allowing yourself to feel sad and frustrated, without feeling guilty about it, is important.
- Seeking spiritual support is helpful for many people.
- If your worry is upsetting to you or your family and lasts for long periods, you should request a referral to a mental health professional who is specially trained to work with cancer patients.

Along with these measures, a doctor may be able to suggest medicines to treat anxiety and depression. Short-term use of these drugs is rarely a problem. It can be just what you need to regroup.

Finding Hope

Hope is a necessary part of everyday life. Hope gets many of us out of bed in the morning and keeps us going throughout the day.

Even if you have advanced cancer, you can still have hopes and dreams. Some of these may have changed since you learned of your cancer. Your hope may be to have a pain-free day. Another hope could be to do something special with a family member. Just talking openly can be a hope that people with cancer and their families can share. There may also be real hope for relief of symptoms and slowing down the growth of the cancer.

Coping with Pain and Discomfort

Advanced illness can cause much discomfort. Dealing with the symptoms is a challenge. Physical pain causes distress to the mind as well. It is essential that you work with your cancer care team to manage your physical symptoms. Severe physical symptoms like pain can make it impossible to have any quality of life. Combining medical treatment with good coping skills is the best way to effectively manage physical symptoms.

Distract yourself

Getting your mind off the pain is always a good idea. It usually hurts more when you are focused on your pain. If you are watching an interesting movie while in pain, you may even forget about it for a while. Visits from friends and family can serve the same purpose.

Get information

Knowing why you have a problem and what you can do about it can relieve stress. Don't be afraid to ask why something is happening.

Take action

Doing something, sometimes anything,. about a problem can help you feel more in control. For example, if the new drug you are taking for your stomach isn't helping, ask to try something else.

Take it one step at a time

It's easy to get overwhelmed if you focus on all the discomforts at once. Tackling one problem at a time makes it seem more possible that all the problems can be helped.

Talk with others

Sometimes, it's a relief just to talk about how discouraged and frustrated you feel about your symptoms. Many people are good listeners and can listen without passing judgment or giving advice.

Express yourself in other ways

For some, talking is not easy. Writing in a journal, painting, or meditating may be other ways for you to express your feelings.

Find your sense of humor

Humor is a tried and true coping skill for rough times. Even when life seems bleak, there is usually something that can lighten the mood and relieve stress.

Practice meditation

By focusing your mind on pleasant scenes, you can direct your attention away from unpleasant feeling and thoughts. This exercise will enable you to get a needed rest, both physically and emotionally.

Relieving Depression

Feeling sad and down at times is normal with illness and the side effects of treatment. But there is room for happiness even with advanced cancer. You don't have to feel down all the time. Depression can be a very serious problem. Therefore, a person who appears to be depressed—regardless of the cause—should be assessed by a trained mental health professional.

About 1 in 4 people with cancer will become depressed. The numbers are higher in those with advanced cancer. All depression can be treated. The symptoms of depression are listed below. Family and friends should watch out for these symptoms. They can encourage the cancer patient to seek professional help.

Symptoms of clinical depression include the following:

- ongoing sad or "empty" mood
- feeling hopeless and helpless
- no interest or pleasure in everyday things
- less energy, feeling tired, being "slowed down"
- trouble sleeping, early waking, or oversleeping
- loss of appetite or overeating
- trouble focusing, remembering, or making decisions
- feeling guilty, worthless, or helpless
- grouchiness
- crying a lot
- ongoing aches and pains for no clear reason

- thoughts of death or suicide; trying to kill yourself

Please see a mental health professional if you have 5 or more of these symptoms for 2 weeks or longer.

Treatment for depression
- medicine
- teaching problem-solving skills
- counseling

People who get treatment for depression are often surprised at how much better they feel. Depression and feelings of sadness can become a way of life. It doesn't have to be that way.

Feeling Less Alone

Depression and feeling alone often go hand in hand. Depression can make you feel the need to withdraw from others. The illness and the demands of treatment sometimes cause you to be alone. People with cancer can end up alone even if they want to be with others. This can happen because of physical problems, lack of transportation, or treatment schedules.

You can feel alone even when you are with well-meaning friends and family. You may have a hard time sharing your feelings about your cancer. Others might be uncomfortable hearing about your illness. This isolation within the company of others can sometimes feel worse than really being alone.

Sometimes a person with cancer needs to ask permission from others to talk more freely. It is also helpful if a friend or family member arranges for others to visit you. Trying to do things outside the home can also make you feel less alone.

Managing Guilt

Both people with cancer and those in their support circle often have feelings of guilt. If you have cancer, you might feel guilty about being ill. These feelings can last even when you know it isn't your fault. Making others aware of your discomfort or telling loved ones that you need their help can make you feel guilty, too.

For the people caring for the patient, guilty feelings can be a daily struggle. Those who are healthy feel guilty about their good health. They often feel bad about not doing enough for their loved one.

Managing feelings of guilt

- Sometimes just talking about the feelings of guilt can help. It can clear the air and ease everyone's conscience. Sharing this common feeling can bring you closer together.
- Letting each other off the hook is helpful. You can tell each other that you know everyone is doing their best.
- For caregivers, sharing the work is important. Friends and family who want to help should be given specific tasks to lighten the main caregiver's load.
- If guilt still persists, it is important that you meet with a trained mental health professional who can help you work through these feelings.

Facing Family Issues

Advanced cancer changes the way family members relate to one another. Families that solve conflict well and support each other do best in dealing with a loved one's cancer. Families who find problem solving hard will have more trouble. You may wish to seek counseling to plan how to best support each other and anticipate problems.

Roles within the family will change. How family members take on new tasks and fill in for the person with cancer affects how they will adjust to losing that person.

For the person with cancer, the changes in family roles can trigger the grief that comes with loss. For example, a bedridden woman may feel anguished about not being the wife and mother she once was. Understanding this and finding ways for her to still contribute and feel included may help both her and her family.

Maintaining Sexual Feelings and Closeness

During advanced illness, a sexual relationship will change. This can be due to physical symptoms, such as fatigue, trouble moving, or pain. It can also come from holding back emotions. Very often sexual desire may decrease, but this does not mean that the need for physical closeness and touching will change. In fact, the need to be held and touched may increase. Talking about feelings and continuing to touch each other can help with feelings of isolation. However, if you have any doubt about whether it is okay to act in a sexual manner or to simply touch, just ask and talk about it. Never ever assume.

Getting Through a Long Illness

Illness that goes on for months or even years puts huge stress on the family. The longer the stress lasts, the more the family is at risk for mental distress. Family members may become exhausted in body and mind. Fatigue added to worry and fear can take a toll. Find ways to get support for the caregivers. Keep asking how everyone is holding up.

Finding Strength in the Spiritual

Spiritual questions are common as a person tries to make sense of both the illness and his or her life. This may be true not only for the person with cancer, but for loved ones as well.

Here are some suggestions for people who may find comfort in spiritual support:

- Help from a spiritual counselor can be timely. He or she can help you find comforting answers to hard questions.
- Religious practices, such as forgiveness or confession, may be reassuring.
- A search for the meaning of suffering can result in a spiritual answer that is comforting.
- Believing in life after death and an end to human suffering on earth is helpful for many.
- Strength through spiritual support and a community of people who are there to help can be priceless to family members.

Facing Death

Anyone with advanced cancer faces the reality that he or she will die. Family members must recognize this too. Even if the person with cancer is doing well, death is a likely part of the future at some point. Thinking about death is frightening and painful for many. Patients and families worry about suffering before death and being alone in death. Sometimes the illness and suffering have gone on for so long that everyone sees death as a relief.

Many people with cancer want to be at home until the end. A long illness and dying at home can be easier with the support of family and medical staff. Often everyone's goal is to help the person with cancer die at home, with loved ones, and with little or no pain.

The American Cancer Society document *Nearing the End of Life* has been written to address questions that patients and family members ask about what to expect during their last 6 months of life. You can get a copy by calling **800-ACS-2345** or visiting our Web site at **www.cancer.org.**

Sources of Support

Caregiver support

People helping to care for the person with cancer need to take care of themselves, too. Taking care of oneself means taking time to do things you enjoy. It also means getting help from others. For more information on this important subject, see the American Cancer Society book *Caregiving: A*

Step-by-Step Resource for Caring for the Person with Cancer at Home.

Support groups

A support group can be a powerful tool for patients and families. Talking with others who are in situations like yours can help ease loneliness. You can talk without being judged. You can also get useful ideas from others that might help you. The American Cancer Society offers many different support group programs in your community.

Choices for Palliative Care

Care aimed at relieving suffering and improving the quality of life is called **palliative care.** The focus of care is the patient and family rather than the disease. Care can be given at home. Some cancer centers actually have special palliative care teams. The team usually has professionals with extra training in cancer and hospice care. Members may include a doctor, chaplain, social worker, nurses, home health aides, physical therapists, a dietitian, pharmacist, and breathing (respiratory) therapist. The palliative care team works with the patient's doctor to develop treatment plans, manage pain and other symptoms, provide emotional support, and help deal with end-of-life issues.

When the Focus Is on Care: Palliative Care and Cancer is a book by the American Cancer Society that discusses many of the questions you may have and provides a list of very helpful resources. Call the American Cancer Society at **800-ACS-2345** or visit our Web site at **www.cancer.org** for more information.

Home care

Home health care is professional health care given in your home. Home care may be right for you if you still need care but no longer need to be in a hospital. A wide range of health and social services can be given at home to people with cancer.

Many home health care agencies offer care and support for patients who choose to stay at home. Home care usually includes regular visits by health care professionals. The family is still responsible for most of the care. It is important to talk with your cancer care team so that you understand what types of care will be needed and how this will affect your family.

Sometimes, the family cannot continue to care for the patient at home. There may not be enough family members to provide all the care needed or the care may be too complex. If this happens, family members may feel guilty, especially if they had promised to care for the patient at home. Recognizing the efforts of family members can help them cope with these feelings. For more information, please see the American Cancer Society document *Home Care*.

Hospice care

Hospice is a program designed to give supportive care near the end of life. The right time for hospice care is when treatment aimed at a cure is no longer helping the patient. Most hospice patients live no more than 6 months. Hospice patients can live longer. Together, the patient, family, and doctor decide when hospice care should begin. Many professionals in the field believe that patients are referred too late. There is much that a hospice program can do for you and your loved ones, even if you are still getting cancer treatment.

Hospice sees death as the natural, final stage of life. It seeks to manage a patient's physical and emotional symptoms. The goal of hospice is that the person's last days be spent with dignity and quality, surrounded by loved ones. Hospice care affirms life and neither hurries nor postpones death. Its focus is on quality of life, rather than length.

Hospice programs offer family-centered care. They involve the patient and family in making decisions. Hospice care is usually given in the home. You might occasionally find hospice care in a hospital or private hospice center. Hospice care can also be made available in some nursing homes.

In a hospice program, a team will usually care for you. The team will have a medical director who is a doctor, a nurse, a nurse's aide, a social worker, and a chaplain. In most cases, your own doctor will also play a role.

There are more than 3,000 hospice programs in the United States. Most of these are designed to provide care in your home. You can find out about hospice in your area by calling HospiceLink at 800-331-1620. Many Web sites can also give you information about hospices (see "Resources" on pages 77–81).

Deciding to begin hospice care can be a tough decision. In general, it means you are giving up any treatment aimed at a cure. An honest talk with your doctor can help you decide if that is the right thing to do. Ask whether any treatment suggested by your doctor offers hope for a cure. If a cure is not possible, will the treatment prolong your life or relieve any of your symptoms?

You should think about hospice if your doctor can't assure you that treatment will meet any of these goals. A hospice program will give you the best chance of controlling your symptoms and keeping the quality of your life. Most experts in palliative care feel that patients enter hospice programs too late to get their full benefit.

Money

It's important to consider money issues when deciding what type of care you will get and where you will get it. Insurance policies differ widely. Check with your insurance company to find out which services are covered. Many insurance companies have a case coordinator as your main contact. This person decides what your benefits cover in your specific case. Most health insurance plans cover hospice care. Many states mandate this. Medicare has a special hospice benefit that not only covers care, but also pays for all medicines. For Medicare information, call the Medicare Helpline at 800-MEDICARE (800-633-4227);

TDD: 877-486-2048. They can explain what Medicare covers and how to qualify.

Serious illnesses often create a need for a lot of money right away. In many states, you can turn death benefits from your life insurance policy into "living benefits." You can get these benefits several ways, such as selling the policy or borrowing against it. For more information, please see the American Cancer Society document *Medical Insurance and Financial Assistance for the Cancer Patient.*

Advance Directives

Everyone has the right to make decisions about his or her own health care. This includes deciding when and if patients want medical treatment to continue or stop. You have the right to accept or refuse treatments, even treatments that will save your life. One way to hold onto your rights is by putting decisions about future health care in writing. This is called an **advance directive.** An advance directive is a legal paper. It can state your wishes about health care choices. It can name someone else to make those choices if you cannot. Doctors follow your advance directive if you can't make medical decisions because of an illness or injury.

Advance directives can only be used for decisions about medical care. Other people cannot use them to control your money or property. Advance directives take effect only when you can't make your own decisions. Others can make health care decisions for you without an advance directive. An advance directive helps you keep some control over these decisions. For more information, please see the American Cancer Society document *Advance Directives.*

Resources

More Information From Your American Cancer Society

We have selected some related information that may also be helpful to you. These materials may be viewed on our Web site or ordered from our toll-free number, **800-ACS-2345.**

Advanced Cancer and Palliative Care Treatment Guidelines for Patients (also available in Spanish)

Advance Directives

American Cancer Society Cancer Survivors' Network (CSN)

Anxiety, Fear and Depression

Bone Metastasis

Breakthrough Cancer Pain: Questions and Answers

Cancer Pain Treatment Guidelines for Patients (also available in Spanish)

Cancer-Related Fatigue and Anemia Treatment Guidelines for Patients (also available in Spanish)

Caring for the Patient with Cancer at Home: A Guide for Patients and Families (also available in Spanish)

Communicating with Friends and Relatives About Your Cancer (also available in Spanish)

Coping with Grief and Loss (also available in Spanish)

Distress Treatment Guidelines for Patients (also available in Spanish)

Family Medical Leave Act

Financial Guidance for Cancer Survivors and Their Families: Advanced Illness

Helping Children When a Family Member Has Cancer: Dealing with a Parent's Terminal Illness

Helping Children When a Family Member Has Cancer: Understanding Psychosocial Support Services

Home Care Agencies (also available in Spanish)

Home Care for the Person with Cancer: A Guide for Patients and Families

Hospice Care (also available in Spanish)

Medical Insurance and Financial Assistance for the Cancer Patient (also available in Spanish)

Nearing the End of Life

Nausea and Vomiting Treatment Guidelines for Patients with Cancer (also available in Spanish)

Nutrition for the Person with Cancer: A Guide for Patients and Families (also available in Spanish)

Pain Control: A Guide for People with Cancer and Their Families (also available in Spanish)

Sexuality and Cancer: For the Man Who Has Cancer and His Partner (also available in Spanish)

Sexuality and Cancer: For the Woman Who Has Cancer and Her Partner (also available in Spanish)

Talking with Your Doctor (also available in Spanish)

Books

The following books are available from the American Cancer Society. Call us at **800-ACS-2345** to ask about costs or to place your order. See other books published by the American Cancer Society at the back of this book.

American Cancer Society's Guide to Pain Control

Caregiving: A Step-By-Step Resource for Caring for the Person with Cancer at Home

Cancer in the Family: Helping Children Cope with a Parent's Illness

When the Focus Is on Care: Palliative Care and Cancer

National Organizations and Web Sites*

The following organizations can provide additional information and resources.*

American Pain Foundation
  Toll-free number: 888-615-7246 (888-615-PAIN)
  Internet address: www.painfoundation.org

CancerCare
  Toll-free number: 800-813-4673 (800-813-HOPE)
  Internet address: www.cancercare.org

Centers for Medicare and Medicaid Services (CMS)
  Toll-free number: 877-267-2323
  Internet address: www.cms.hhs.gov

Family and Medical Leave Act
  Toll-free number: 866-487-9243 (866-4USWAGE)
  Internet address: www.dol.gov/esa/whd/fmla

Family Caregiver Alliance
  Toll-free number: 800-445-8106
  Internet address: www.caregiver.org

Hospice Association of America
  Telephone: 202-546-4759
  Internet address: www.hospice-america.org

Hospice Education Institute/HospiceLink
  Toll-free number: 800-331-1620
  Internet address: www.hospiceworld.org

Hospice Foundation of America
  Toll-free number: 800-854-3402
  Internet address: www.hospicefoundation.org

Hospice Net
  Internet address: www.hospicenet.org
  This organization works only through the
  Internet.

National Alliance for Caregiving (NAC)
  Internet address: www.caregiving.org

National Association for Home Care and Hospice (NAHC)
  Telephone: 202-547-7424
  Internet address: www.nahc.org

National Hospice and Palliative Care Organization
  Toll-free number: 800-658-8898
  Internet address: www.nhpco.org

Substance Abuse and Mental Health Services
  Administration (SAMHSA)
  Mental Health Information Center
  Toll-free number: 800-789-2647

Suicide Prevention Hotline
  Toll-free number: 800-273-TALK (8255)
  Internet address: www.samhsa.gov

*Inclusion on this list does not imply endorsement by the American Cancer Society.

The American Cancer Society is happy to address almost any cancer-related topic. If you have any more questions, please call us at **800-ACS-2345** at any time, 24 hours a day.

References

Berger A, Portenoy RK, Weissman DE, eds. *Principles and Practice of Supportive Oncology.* Philadelphia, PA: Lippincott-Raven; 1998.

Bruera E, Kim HN. Cancer Pain. *JAMA.* 2003;290:2476–2479.

Groenwald SL, Frogge MH, Goodman M, Yarbro CH, eds. *Cancer Symptom Management*. Boston, MA: Jones & Bartlett; 1996.

Liotta LA, Kohn EC. Invasion and metastasis. In: Kufe DW, Pollock RE, Weichselbaum RR, Bast RC, Gansler TS, Holland JF, Frei E, eds. *Cancer Medicine 6*. Hamilton, Ontario: BC Decker; 2003:151–160.

Glossary

advanced cancer: a general term describing stages of cancer in which the disease has spread from the primary site to other parts of the body. When the cancer has spread only to the surrounding areas, it is called locally advanced. If it has spread to distant parts of the body, it is called metastatic.

advance directive: a legal document that tells the doctor and family what a person wants for future medical care, including whether to start or when to stop life-sustaining treatment.

alternative medicine: an unproven medication or therapy that is recommended instead of standard (proven) therapy. Some alternative therapies have dangerous or even life-threatening side effects. With others, the main danger is that the patient may lose the opportunity to benefit from standard therapy. The American Cancer Society recommends that patients considering the use of any alternative or complementary therapy discuss this with their health care team. *See also* complementary medicine.

androgen (AN-dro-jen): any male sex hormone. The major androgen is testosterone.

anemia (uh-NEEM-ee-uh): low red blood cell count.

anesthesia (an-es-THEE-zhuh): the loss of feeling or sensation as a result of drugs or gases. General anesthesia causes loss of consciousness (puts you to sleep). Local or regional anesthesia numbs only a certain area.

angiogenesis (an-jee-o-JEN-uh-sis): the formation of new blood vessels. Some cancer treatments work by blocking angiogenesis, thus preventing blood from reaching the tumor.

antibiotic: a drug used to kill organisms that cause disease. Antibiotics may be made by living organisms or they may be created in the lab. Since some cancer treatments can reduce the body's ability to fight off infection, antibiotics may be used to treat or prevent these infections.

antigen (AN-tuh-jen): a substance that causes the body's immune system to react. This reaction often involves production of antibodies. For example, the immune system's response to antigens that are part of bacteria and viruses helps people resist infections. Cancer cells have certain antigens that can be found by laboratory tests. They are important in cancer diagnosis and in watching response to treatment. Other cancer cell antigens play a role in immune reactions that may help the body's resistance against cancer.

ascites (uh-SY-teez): abnormal buildup of fluid in the abdomen that may cause swelling. In late-stage cancer, tumor cells may be found in the fluid in the abdomen. Ascites also occurs in patients with liver disease.

aspiration (as-per-AY-shun): the accidental breathing in of food or fluid into the lungs. Also, removal of fluid or tissues through a needle. *See also* fine needle biopsy.

biopsy (BUY-op-see): the removal of a sample of tissue to see whether cancer cells are present. There are several kinds of biopsies. In some, a very thin needle is used to draw fluid and cells from a lump. In a **core needle biopsy,** a larger needle is used to remove more tissue. *See* core needle biopsy, fine needle biopsy, CT–guided needle biopsy, bone marrow biopsy, incisional biopsy.

bisphosphonates: drugs that are sometimes given to cancer patients whose disease has spread to the bones. When injected into a vein or taken by mouth, bisphosphonates can slow the breakdown of bone, lower the rate of bone fractures, and treat bone pain.

bone marrow: the soft tissue in the hollow of flat bones of the body that produces new blood cells.

bone marrow biopsy: a procedure in which a needle is placed into the cavity of a bone, usually the hip or breast bone, to remove a small amount of bone marrow for examination under a microscope.

bone scan: an imaging method that gives important information about the bones, including the location of cancer that may have spread to the bones. It can be done as an outpatient procedure and is painless, except for the needle stick when a low-dose radioactive substance is injected into a vein. Special pictures are taken to see where the radioactivity collects, pointing to an abnormality. *See also* radionuclide bone scan, imaging tests.

brachytherapy (brake-ee-THER-uh-pee): internal radiation treatment given by placing radioactive material directly into the tumor or close to it. Also called interstitial radiation therapy or seed implantation. *See* internal radiation therapy. *Compare with* external beam radiation therapy.

cancer: cancer is not just one disease but a group of diseases. All forms of cancer cause cells in the body to change and grow out of control. Most types of cancer cells form a lump or mass called a tumor. The tumor can invade and destroy healthy tissue. Cells from the tumor can break away and travel to other parts of the body, where they can continue to grow. This spreading process is called metastasis. When cancer spreads, it is still named after the part of the body where it started. For example, if breast cancer spreads to the lungs, it is still breast cancer, not lung cancer.

Some cancers, such as blood cancers, do not form a tumor. Not all tumors are cancer. A tumor that is not cancer is called benign. Benign tumors do not grow and spread the way cancer does. They are usually not a threat to life. Another word for cancerous is malignant.

cancer care team: the group of health care professionals who work together to find, treat, and care for people with cancer. The cancer care team may include the following and others: primary care physicians, pathologists, oncology specialists (medical oncologist, radiation oncologist), surgeons (including surgical specialists such as urologists, gynecologists, neurosurgeons, etc.), nurses, nurse practitioners, oncology nurse specialists, and oncology social workers. Whether the team is linked formally or informally, there is usually one person who takes the job of coordinating the team.

cancer cell: a cell that divides and reproduces abnormally and has the potential to spread throughout the body, crowding out normal cells and tissue.

cancer of unknown primary: the diagnosis when metastatic cancer is found, but the place where the cancer began (the primary site) cannot be found.

cancer-related fatigue (fuh-TEEG): an unusual and persistent sense of tiredness that can occur with cancer or cancer treatments. It can be overwhelming, last a long time, and interfere with everyday life. Rest does not always relieve it.

capillary: the smallest type of blood vessel. A capillary connects a small artery to a small vein to form a network of blood vessels in almost all parts of the body. The wall of a capillary is thin and leaky, and capillaries are involved in the exchange of fluids and gases between tissues and the blood.

carcinoembryonic antigen (kahr-si-no-em-bre-AHN-ik AN-tuh-jen) (CEA): a substance normally found in fetal tissue. If found in an adult, it may suggest that a cancer, especially one starting in the digestive system, may be present. Tests for this substance may help in finding out if a colorectal cancer has recurred after treatment. The test is not helpful for screening for colorectal cancer because of the large number of false positives and false negatives. *See* antigen, tumor marker, screening.

cauterization (kaw-teh-ri-ZAY-shun): destruction of tissue with a hot or cold instrument, an electrical current, or a chemical that burns or dissolves the tissue. This process may be used to kill certain types of small tumors or to seal off blood vessels to stop bleeding.

CEA: *see* carcinoembryonic antigen.

cell: the basic unit of which all living things are made. Cells replace themselves by splitting and forming new cells (*mitosis*). The processes that control the formation of new cells and the death of old cells are disrupted in cancer.

chemotherapy (key-mo-THER-uh-pee): treatment with drugs to destroy cancer cells. Chemotherapy is often used, either alone or with surgery or radiation, to treat cancer that has spread or come back (recurred), or when there is a strong chance that it could recur.

clinical trials: research studies to test new drugs or other treatments to compare current, standard treatments with others that may be better. Before a new treatment is used on people, it is studied in the lab. If lab studies suggest the treatment will work, the next step is to test its value for patients. These human studies are called clinical trials. The main questions the researchers want to answer are—
- Does this treatment work?
- Does it work better than what we're now using?
- What side effects does it cause?
- Do the benefits outweigh the risks?
- Which patients are most likely to find this treatment helpful?

colostomy (kuh-LAHS-tuh-me): a procedure in which the end of the colon is attached to an opening created in the abdominal wall to get rid of body waste (stool). A colostomy is sometimes needed after surgery for cancer of the rectum. People with colon cancer sometimes have a temporary colostomy, but they rarely need a permanent one.

complementary medicine: treatment used in addition to standard therapy. Some complementary therapies may help relieve certain symptoms of cancer, relieve side effects of standard cancer therapy, or improve a patient's sense of well-being. The American Cancer Society recommends that patients considering the use of any alternative or complementary therapy discuss this with their health care team, since many of these treatments are unproven and some can be harmful. *See also* alternative medicine.

computed tomography (toh-MAHG-ruh-fee): an imaging test in which many x-rays are taken from different angles of a part of the body. These images are combined by a computer to produce cross-sectional pictures of internal organs. Except for the injection of a dye (needed in some but not all cases), this is a painless procedure that can be done in an outpatient clinic. It is often referred to as a "CT" or "CAT" scan.

contrast dye: any material used in imaging studies such as x-rays, MRI and CT scans to help outline the body parts being examined. These may be injected or ingested (drunk). Also called dye, radiocontrast dye, radiocontrast medium. *See also* imaging tests.

control group: in research or clinical trials, the group that does not receive the treatment being tested. The group may get a placebo or sham treatment, or it may receive standard therapy. Also called the comparison group. *See also* clinical trials.

core needle biopsy: removal of fluid, cells, or tissue with a needle for examination under a microscope. A core needle biopsy uses a thicker needle than that used in fine needle aspirates to remove a cylindrical sample of tissue from a tumor. *See also* fine needle biopsy.

CT–guided needle biopsy: a procedure that uses special x-rays to locate a mass, while the radiologist advances a biopsy needle toward it. The images are repeated until the doctor is sure the needle is in the tumor or mass. A small sample of tissue is then taken from the mass to be examined under the microscope. *See also* biopsy.

CT scan or **CAT scan:** *see* computed tomography.

cytokine (SIGHT-o-kine): a product of cells of the immune system that may stimulate immunity and cause the regression of some cancers.

dehydration: a condition that results from excessive loss of water.

distant recurrence: cancer that has spread far from its original location or primary site to distant organs or lymph nodes. Sometimes called **distant metastases.** *See also* primary site, recurrence; *compare with* local or localized cancer.

dyspnea: breathlessness or shortness of breath.

ECM: *see* extracellular matrix.

embolization (em-buh-luh-ZAY-shun): a type of treatment that reduces the blood supply to the cancer by the injection of materials to plug up the artery that supplies blood to the tumor.

enzyme: a protein that speeds up chemical reactions in the body.

external beam radiation therapy (EBRT): radiation that is focused from a source outside the body on the area affected by the cancer. It is much like getting a diagnostic x-ray, but for a longer time. *Compare with* brachytherapy, internal radiation therapy.

extracellular matrix (ECM): any material produced by cells and excreted to the extracellular space within the tissues. ECM is like the mortar holding bricks together to form the walls of buildings. It serves to hold tissues together, and its form and composition help determine tissue characteristics.

fatigue (fuh-TEEG): a common symptom during cancer treatment, a bone-weary exhaustion that doesn't get better with rest. For some, this can last for some time after treatment. *See also* cancer-related fatigue.

FDA: *see* U.S. Food and Drug Administration.

fine needle biopsy: a procedure in which a thin needle is used to draw up (aspirate) samples for examination under a microscope. *See also* biopsy.

grade: the grade of a cancer reflects how abnormal it looks under the microscope. There are several grading systems for different types of cancers. Each grading system divides cancer into those with the greatest abnormality, the least abnormality, and those in between.

Grading is done by a pathologist who examines the tissue from the biopsy. It is important because cancers with more abnormal-appearing cells tend to grow and spread more quickly and have a worse prognosis (outlook). *See also* pathologist, prognosis.

hormone: a chemical substance released into the body by the endocrine glands such as the thyroid, adrenal, or ovaries. Hormones travel through the bloodstream and set in motion various body functions. Testosterone and estrogen are examples of male and female hormones.

hormone therapy: treatment with hormones, with drugs that interfere with hormone production or hormone action, or the surgical removal of hormone-producing glands. Hormone therapy may kill cancer cells or slow their growth. *See also* hormone.

hospice: a special kind of care for people in the final phase of illness and their families and caregivers. The care may take place in the patient's home or in a homelike facility.

hot spots: areas of diseased bone that show up on bone scans. The hot spots can be bone metastasis, but they may also represent arthritis, infection, or other bone diseases.

hypercalcemia (hy-per-kal-SEE-mee-uh): a high calcium level in the blood, sometimes due to cancer cells causing the release of calcium from bones.

imaging tests: methods used to produce pictures of internal body structures. Some imaging methods used to help diagnose or stage cancer are x-rays, CT scans, magnetic resonance imaging (MRI), and ultrasound.

incisional biopsy: a surgical procedure in which tissue is removed and examined by a pathologist. The pathologist may study the tissue under a microscope or perform other tests. When an entire lump or suspicious area is removed, the procedure is called an excisional biopsy. When a sample of tissue or fluid is removed with a needle, the procedure is called a needle biopsy, core biopsy, or fine-needle biopsy (aspiration).

informed consent: a legal document that explains a course of treatment, the risks, benefits, and possible alternatives; the process by which patients agree to treatment.

internal radiation therapy: treatment involving implantation of a radioactive substance. *See* brachytherapy. *Compare with* external beam radiation therapy.

intravenous (in-tra-VEEN-us) (IV) line: a method of supplying fluids and medications by using a needle or a thin tube inserted in a vein.

jaundice (JAWN-dis): a condition in which the skin and the whites of the eyes become yellow, urine darkens, and the color of the stool becomes lighter than normal. Jaundice occurs when the liver is not working properly or when a bile duct is blocked.

leukemia (loo-KEY-me-uh): cancer of the blood or blood-forming organs. People with leukemia often have a noticeable increase in white blood cells (leukocytes).

living will: a legal document that allows a person to decide what to do if he or she becomes unable to make health care decisions; a type of advance directive. *See also* advance directive.

local or **localized cancer:** a cancer that is confined to the organ where it started; that is, it has not spread to distant parts of the body.

local recurrence: *see* recurrence.

lymph (limf): clear fluid that flows through the lymphatic vessels and contains cells known as lymphocytes. These cells are important in fighting infections and may also have a role in fighting cancer. *See also* lymphatic system, lymph nodes, lymphocyte, lymphadenectomy.

lymphadenectomy (lim-fad-uh-NECK-tuh-me): surgical removal of one or more lymph nodes. After removal, the lymph nodes are examined by microscope to see if cancer has spread. Also called lymph node dissection. *See also* lymphatic system, lymph, lymph nodes, lymphocyte.

lymphatic system: the tissues and organs (including lymph nodes, spleen, thymus, and bone marrow) that produce and store lymphocytes (cells that fight infection) and the channels that carry the lymph fluid. The entire lymphatic system is an important part of the body's immune system. Invasive cancers sometimes penetrate the lymphatic vessels (channels) and spread (metastasize) to lymph nodes. *See also* lymph, lymph nodes, lymphocyte, lymphadenectomy.

lymph nodes: small bean-shaped collections of immune system tissue such as lymphocytes, found along lymphatic vessels. They remove cell waste, germs, and other harmful substances from lymph. They help fight infections and also have a role in fighting cancer, although cancers sometimes spread through them. Also called lymph glands. *See also* lymph, lymphatic system, lymphadenectomy.

lymphocyte (LIM-fo-sight): a type of white blood cell that helps the body fight infection.

lymphoma (lim-FOAM-uh): a cancer of the lymphatic system, a network of thin vessels and nodes throughout the body. Its function is to fight infection. Lymphoma involves a type of white blood cells called lymphocytes. The 2 main types of lymphoma are Hodgkin disease and non-Hodgkin lymphoma. The treatment methods for these 2 types of lymphomas are very different.

magnetic resonance imaging (MRI): a method of taking pictures of the inside of the body. Instead of using x-rays, MRI uses a powerful magnet to send radio waves through the body. The images appear on a computer screen, as well as on film. Like x-rays, the procedure is physically painless, but some people may feel confined inside the MRI machine.

malignant (muh-LIG-nunt) tumor: a mass of cancer cells that may invade surrounding tissues or spread (metastasize) to distant areas of the body. *See also* tumor, metastasis.

metastasis (meh-TAS-tuh-sis): cancer cells that have spread to one or more sites elsewhere in the body, often by way of the lymphatic system or bloodstream. **Regional metastasis** is cancer that has spread to the lymph nodes, tissues, or organs close to the primary site. **Distant metastasis** is cancer that has spread to organs or tissues that are farther away (such as when prostate cancer spreads to the bones, lungs, or liver). The plural of this word is metastases. *See also* primary site, lymph nodes, lymphatic system, local or localized cancer, regional recurrence or regional spread.

metastasize (meh-TAS-tuh-size): the spread of cancer cells to one or more sites elsewhere in the body, often by way of the lymphatic system or bloodstream. *See also* metastasis, lymphatic system.

metastatic (met-uh-STAT-ick) cancer: a way to describe cancer that has spread from the primary site (where it started) to other structures or organs, nearby or far away (distant). *See also* primary site, metastasis.

metastatic recurrence: *see* recurrence.

MRI: *see* magnetic resonance imaging.

needle aspiration (as-puh-RAY-shun): a type of needle biopsy. Removal of fluid from a cyst or cells from a tumor. In this procedure, a needle is used to reach the cyst or tumor, and with suction, draw up (aspirate) samples for examination under a microscope. If the needle is thin, the procedure is called a fine needle aspiration or FNA. *See also* biopsy.

needle biopsy: removal of fluid, cells, or tissue with a needle for examination under a microscope. There are 2 types: **fine needle aspiration** (FNA) and **core biopsy.** FNA uses a thin needle to draw up (aspirate) fluid or small tissue fragments from a cyst or tumor. A core needle biopsy uses a thicker needle to remove a cylindrical sample of tissue from a tumor.

oncologist (on-CAHL-uh-jist): a doctor with special training in the diagnosis and treatment of cancer.

osteolytic metastases: the spread of cancer cells to the bone, which causes the bone to break down.

palliative care: *see* palliative treatment.

palliative (PAL-ee-uh-tiv) radiation: *see* palliative treatment.

palliative (PAL-ee-uh-tiv) treatment: treatment that relieves symptoms, such as pain, but is not expected to cure the disease. Its main purpose is to improve the patient's quality of life. Sometimes chemotherapy and radiation are used in this way.

pathologist (path-AHL-o-jist): a doctor who specializes in diagnosis and classification of diseases by laboratory tests such as examining cells under a microscope. The pathologist determines whether a tumor is benign or cancerous and, if cancerous, the exact cell type and grade.

pericardium: the fibroserous sac that surrounds the heart and the roots of the great vessels.

PET: *see* positron emission tomography.

platelet (PLATE-uh-let): a part of the blood that plugs up holes in blood vessels after an injury. Chemotherapy can cause a drop in the platelet count, a condition called thrombocytopenia that carries a risk of excessive bleeding.

positron emission tomography (PAHS-ih-trahn ee-MISH-uhn toh-MAHG-ruh-fee) (PET): a PET scan creates an image of the body (or of biochemical events) after the injection of a very low dose of a radioactive form of a substance such as glucose (sugar). The scan computes the rate at which the tumor is using the sugar. In general, high-grade tumors use more sugar than normal and low-grade tumors use less. PET scans are especially useful in taking images of the brain, although they are becoming more widely used to find the spread of cancer of the breast, colon, rectum, ovary, or lung. PET scans may also be used to see how well the tumor is responding to treatment.

primary site: the place where cancer begins. Primary cancer is usually named after the organ in which it starts.

For example, cancer that starts in the breast is always breast cancer even if it spreads (metastasizes) to other organs such as bones or lungs.

prognosis (prog-NO-sis): a prediction of the course of disease; the outlook for the chances of survival.

prostate-specific antigen (PSA): a substance produced by the prostate that may be found in an increased amount in the blood of men who have prostate cancer. *See also* antigen, prostate-specific antigen test.

prostate-specific antigen test: a blood test that measures the level of prostate-specific antigen (PSA), a substance produced by the prostate and some other tissues in the body. Increased levels of PSA may be a sign of prostate cancer.

PSA: *see* prostate-specific antigen, prostate-specific antigen test.

psychiatrist: a medical doctor specializing in mental health and behavioral disorders. Psychiatrists provide counseling and can also prescribe medications.

psychologist: a health professional who assesses a person's mental and emotional status and provides counseling.

quality of life: overall enjoyment of life, which includes a person's sense of well-being and ability to do the things that are important to him or her.

radiation therapy: treatment with high-energy rays (such as x-rays) to kill or shrink cancer cells. The radiation may come from outside of the body (external radiation) or from radioactive materials placed directly in the tumor (brachytherapy or internal radiation). Radiation therapy may be used as the main treatment for a cancer, to reduce the size of a cancer before surgery, or to destroy any remaining cancer cells after surgery. In advanced cancer cases, it may also be used as palliative treatment. *See also* external beam radiation therapy, brachytherapy, palliative treatment.

radiologist: a doctor with special training in diagnosis of diseases by interpreting x-rays and other types of diagnostic imaging studies; for example, CT and MRI scans.

radionuclide (ray-dee-oh-NOO-klide) bone scan: an imaging test that uses a small amount of radioactive contrast material. Given in the vein, the radioactive material settles in "hot spots," areas of bone to which the cancer may have spread, and shows up in the picture. *See also* imaging tests.

recurrence: the return of cancer after treatment. **Local** recurrence means that the cancer has come back at the same place as the original cancer. **Regional** recurrence means that the cancer has come back after treatment in the lymph nodes near the primary site. **Distant** recurrence, also known as **metastatic recurrence,** is when cancer metastasizes *after* treatment to distant organs or tissues (such as the lungs, liver, bone marrow, or brain). *See also* primary site, metastasis, metastasize, relapse.

red blood cells: blood cells that contain hemoglobin, the substance that carries oxygen to all of the cells of the body. *See also* anemia.

regional recurrence or regional spread: the spread of cancer from its original site to nearby areas such as lymph nodes, but not to distant sites. *See also* metastasis, recurrence.

relapse: reappearance of cancer after a disease-free period. *See also* recurrence.

remission: complete or partial disappearance of the signs and symptoms of cancer in response to treatment; the period during which a disease is under control. A remission may not be a cure.

scan: a study using either x-rays or radioactive isotopes to produce images of internal body organs.

screening: the search for disease, such as cancer, in people without symptoms. For example, screening measures for prostate cancer include digital rectal examination and the PSA blood test; for breast cancer, mammograms and clinical breast exams. Screening may refer to coordinated programs in large groups of people.

side effects: unwanted effects of treatment such as hair loss caused by chemotherapy, and fatigue caused by radiation therapy.

sign: an observable physical change caused by an illness. *Compare to* symptom.

social worker: a health professional who helps people find community resources and provides counseling and guidance to assist with issues such as insurance coverage and nursing home placement.

symptom: a change in the body caused by an illness, as described by the person experiencing it. *Compare to* sign.

systemic therapy: treatment that reaches and affects cells throughout the body; for example, chemotherapy. *See also* hormone therapy.

technetium diphosphonate: the radioactive substance that is usually injected into a patient's vein during a radionuclide bone scan. The radioactive material settles in "hot spots," areas of bone to which the cancer may have spread, and shows up in the picture. *See also* radionuclide bone scan, hot spots.

tissue: a collection of cells, united to perform a particular function.

tumor: an abnormal lump or mass of tissue. Tumors can be benign (noncancerous) or malignant (cancerous).

tumor marker: a substance produced by cancer cells and sometimes normal cells. Tumor markers are not very useful for cancer screening because other body tissues not related to a cancer can produce the substance. But tumor markers may be very useful in monitoring for response to treatment when a cancer is diagnosed or for a recurrence. Tumor markers include CA 125 (ovarian cancer), CEA (GI tract cancers), and PSA (prostate cancer).

ultrasound: an imaging method in which high-frequency sound waves are used to outline a part of the body. The sound wave echoes are picked up and displayed on a television screen. Also called ultrasonography.

U.S. Food and Drug Administration (FDA): an agency of the United States Department of Health and Human Services. The FDA is responsible for drugs, biological medical products, blood products, medical devices, and radiation-emitting devices, along with other products.

x-ray: one form of radiation that can be used at low levels to produce an image of the body on film or at high levels to destroy cancer cells.

Index

Books Published
by the American Cancer Society

Available everywhere books are sold and online at
www.cancer.org/bookstore

Cancer Information

General

The Cancer Atlas (available in English, Spanish, French, Chinese)

Cancer: What Causes It, What Doesn't

The Tobacco Atlas, Second Edition (available in English, Spanish, French)

Information for People with Cancer

Site-Specific

ACS's Complete Guide to Colorectal Cancer

ACS's Complete Guide to Prostate Cancer

Breast Cancer Clear & Simple: All Your Questions Answered

QuickFACTS™ Bone Metastasis

QuickFACTS™ Lung Cancer

QuickFACTS™ Prostate Cancer

Praise for *QuickFACTS™ Lung Cancer:*
"The ACS has achieved its goal of providing overviews
that tackle need-to-know issues and supply references for
additional follow-up information as desired.
Recommended."
—Library Journal

Symptoms and Side Effects

ACS's Guide to Pain Control, Revised Edition

Eating Well, Staying Well During and After Cancer

Lymphedema: Understanding and Managing Lymphedema After Cancer Treatment

Support for Families and Caregivers

Cancer in the Family: Helping Children Cope with a Parent's Illness

Caregiving: A Step-by-Step Resource for Caring for the Person with Cancer at Home, Revised Edition

Couples Confronting Cancer: Keeping Your Relationship Strong

Get Better! Communication Cards for Kids & Adults (bilingual communication cards)

Social Work in Oncology: Supporting Survivors, Families, and Caregivers

When the Focus Is on Care: Palliative Care and Cancer

Help for Children

Because . . . Someone I Love Has Cancer: Kids' Activity Book (5 twist-up crayons included)

Mom and the Polka-Dot Boo-Boo

Our Dad Is Getting Better

Our Mom Has Cancer (available in hard cover and paperback)

Our Mom Is Getting Better

Health Books for Children

Healthy Air: A Read-Along Coloring & Activity Book (25 per pack; Tobacco avoidance)

Healthy Bodies: A Read-Along Coloring & Activity Book (25 per pack; Physical activity)

Healthy Food: A Read-Along Coloring & Activity Book (25 per pack; Nutrition)

Healthy Me: A Read-Along Coloring & Activity Book

Kids' First Cookbook: Delicious-Nutritious Treats to Make Yourself!

Tools for the Health Conscious

ACS's Healthy Eating Cookbook, Third Edition

Celebrate! Healthy Entertaining for Any Occasion

Good for You! Reducing Your Risk of Developing Cancer

The Great American Eat-Right Cookbook

Kicking Butts: Quit Smoking and Take Charge of Your Health

National Health Education Standards: Achieving Excellence, Second Edition (available in paperback and on CD-ROM)

Inspirational Survivor Stories

Angels & Monsters: A child's eye view of cancer

Crossing Divides: A Couple's Story of Cancer, Hope, and Hiking Montana's Continental Divide

I Can Survive (Illustrated)*

*A "Mom's Choice Awards" Finalist! (2007)